INSTANT PAIN CONTROL

A fully illustrated guide that explains a simple technique for treating muscle aches and pains at their source.

INSTANT PAIN CONTROL

Using the Body's Trigger Points

by

Leon Chaitow
N.D., D.O.

Line drawings by Bevil Roberts
Photographs by Paul Turner

THORSONS PUBLISHING GROUP

First published 1981
This edition published 1984

British Library Cataloguing in Publication Data

Chaitow, Leon
Instant pain control. — 2nd ed.
1. Manipulation (Therapeutics)
2. Self-care, Health
I. Title
615.8'22   RM724

ISBN 0-7225-0977-4

Published by Thorsons Publishers Limited,
Wellingborough, Northamptonshire, NN8 2RQ, England

Printed in Great Britain by Richard Clay Limited,
Bungay, Suffolk

5 7 9 10 8 6 4

CONTENTS

I dedicate this book to the memory of Stavros Metallinos, with affection.

INTRODUCTION

The framework of the human body is held together by a substance known as *fascia*. This is a connective tissue which envelops the muscles, nerves and blood vessels and which gives cohesion and order to the myriad components of the body. It allows movement between adjacent structures and reduces the effects of pressure and friction. It is rich in nerve endings and has the ability to contract and stretch elastically. It is used by the muscles in their attachment to bones. Because of its many functions, fascia is a vital component in the biomechanical (and biochemical) efficiency of the body.

Postural, emotional and mechanical stress or injury can produce changes in the fascia which may become chronic. A number of other factors might produce changes in these tissues, including infection, excessive heat or cold, allergic inflammatory reactions, inherited factors and arthritic changes in joints. Thus, many possible causes exist for changes in this all-pervasive soft tissue. When such changes take place a varying degree of local tissue tension and contraction is present and distinct localized areas within these tissues become sensitive to pressure.

When pressure on such a sensitive point produces pain in an area some distance from the point itself, then it is called a *trigger area* or *trigger point*. The distant area of pain is known as the *referred area* or the *target area*.

Trigger Point Effects
The disturbing effects of such trigger points go far beyond the simple production and maintenance of pain. A whole range of symptoms can be produced by triggers via their effect on the nervous system, circulatory function and hormonal balance.

Dr Janet Travell, who has pioneered the work on trigger points (myofascial triggers), maintains that the high intensity of nerve impulses from an active trigger can produce, by reflex, vaso-constriction, cutting down the blood supply to specific areas of the brain, spinal cord and nervous system, thus producing any of a wide range of symptoms, capable of affecting almost any part of the body. Such symptoms as disordered vision, disordered respiration, muscle weakness and skin sensitivity are reported by her as resulting from trigger areas in specific muscles.

Dr R. Gutstein has also shown that trigger points (he calls them 'myodysneuric points') can affect vision. He also lists the following possible symptoms from active triggers: pain, numbness, itching, over-sensitivity to normal stimuli, spasm, twitching, weakness and trembling of muscles, tension or weakness of muscle connected with blood vessels, over- or under-secretion of glands (internal, skin etc.). He talks of patterns of abnormality including coldness, paleness, redness of tissues as well as many of the vague menopausal symptoms such as 'flushes' disappearing when triggers in the neck, chest and upper body are treated and removed.

The secretion and, therefore, the texture of skin and hair are altered for the better, especially when triggers in the neck and between the shoulder blades are removed. Similar triggers also affected the tendency to the over- or under-production of sweat. Gutstein quotes a number of practitioners who have improved digestive problems by removing triggers in the chest and abdominal regions. Among these symptoms were spasm of the pylorus, bad breath, heartburn, vomiting, nausea, distension, nervous diarrhoea and constipation.

Trigger and Target
In the main, however, the symptoms dealt with are those of pain and discomfort with consequent limitation of use. Triggers are dealt with in a variety of ways. Some practitioners inject these with drugs such as procaine or xylocaine, others actually remove them surgically. The majority of those in the field of manipulative medicine use techniques of pressure and stretching of the affected area, often combined with the use of chilling techniques, in order to break the vicious cycle created by the trigger point.

These latter techniques are also suitable for the individual to use as first-aid measures, primarily in dealing with the painful symptoms created by triggers. Triggers are always localized areas of deep tenderness and increased resistance to pressure. That is, the tissue feels firmer or harder than the surrounding tissue, and is sensitive to deep pressure. If it is active, pressure on a trigger will often produce twitching or a sort of shivering in the muscles. If the pressure is maintained for a few seconds, pain will be felt in a predictable area. The target area will always be the same for a particular trigger in everyone. Thus, the active trigger in the sternomastoid muscle (Section 1) will always produce pain round the ear, on the cheek, forehead etc. If the trigger is silent or dormant, it may not actually be producing symptoms, but will produce pain in the target area if strong pressure is maintained on it.

Dr J. Mennell states that any muscle that can reach and maintain a normal resting length is free of trigger points. One that cannot is usually a source of pain. He has shown that, in order to eliminate a trigger, it is necessary, after (or during) the main treatment (pressure, chilling etc.), to stretch the muscle fully. He describes the trigger points as localized, palpable spots of deep hypersensitivity, from which noxious (harmful) impulses bombard the central nervous system to give rise to referred pain and other symptoms.

Neuro-muscular Technique
Osteopaths in the United Kingdom use a method of soft tissue manipulation called Neuromuscular Technique which was developed by the great naturopathic pioneer, Stanley Lief. Further refinement of the technique was made by his cousin, my uncle, Boris Chaitow. This technique employs deep-pressure and stretching methods which are highly efficient in removing trigger points. These methods are described in detail in my book *Neuro-muscular Technique* (Thorsons, 1980), but a simple home treatment method will be explained in this book. *This is suitable for self treatment, or treatment of a member of one's family, for first-aid only.*

Rules to be Observed
In order to avoid the side-effects or harmful consequences the following rules should be strictly followed:

1. Only treat trigger points in order to ease pain. Other symptoms may or may not be the result of trigger activity and a competent diagnosis should be obtained.

2. Only treat painful symptoms from a 'first-aid' viewpoint. If the pain does not ease, or eases but returns, then consult a qualified osteopath or chiropractor as there may be mechanical (joint or bone) factors maintaining the trigger, and these require expert attention.

3. Never treat on or near a swelling, lump or inflamed (i.e. red) area.

4. Never treat on a scar, wart, mole or varicose vein.

5. Never treat on a woman's breast.

6. A pregnant woman should never be treated by these methods.

7. If a diagnosis of rheumatoid arthritis or cancer exists then take professional advice before using these methods.

8. Trigger points are often the same as acupuncture points but never stick a needle into these points.

9. Do not overtreat. Observe the methods advocated. Because a certain amount of treatment is helpful, it does not follow that even more is better.

10. Try to discover the deeper causes of the problem. If the triggers are the long-term result of postural stress (typists, dentists, hairdressers etc.), or emotional stress or nutritional inadequacy (e.g. excessive refined carbo-hydrates such as white sugar and white flour products can result in vitamin and mineral deficiency and consequent muscular and nervous dysfunction), then the causes must be dealt with if a quick return of symptoms is to be avoided. Learn postural efficiency, relaxation techniques and adopt wholefood eating habits.

Treatment of Trigger Points

If pain exists in an area listed in the *Index of Symptoms* or shown in any of the illustrations, then search the appropriate trigger area (given in the section or sections indicated by the index) for a sensitive spot. Where more than one section is indicated, you should look up the detailed list of symptoms given in each to discover the position of the trigger responsible for your particular *group* of symptoms. To probe for a sensitive area, use the tip of the thumb or index finger. Press slowly and deeply until an area of sensitivity is found. This should receive sustained pressure for up to ten seconds to see if a referred pain is felt in the target area. This would be an intensification of the existing pain.

If a trigger lies in the neck or upper shoulder muscles (scalenes, sternomastoid and upper trapezius) then pressure of this sort should be avoided and the trigger should be sought by squeezing the muscle between the tips of the thumb and index finger.

Once located and identified as an active trigger, the point should receive up to one minute of sustained or intermittent pressure (or squeezing). The amount of pressure should be great enough to produce the referred effect. If this is intensely uncomfortable, then apply intermittent pressure i.e. five seconds deep, five seconds less deep (easing off by about 25 per cent) and so on until a minute has elapsed. If, during either of these pressure-treatments, the pain in the target area begins to ease significantly, then stop the pressure treatment.

After pressure (or squeezing) treatment, chilling must be applied (see instructions below) during and after which the muscles of the area must be stretched to their physiological limit. Guidance on the stretching is given in the text for each trigger. If pain diminishes after such treatment, do not apply further treatment that day. If there is some improvement or if symptoms return as strongly as before, despite repeated treatment, then there may be causative factors maintaining the triggers which require expert attention. A qualified osteopath or chiropractor should be consulted.

Note. The pressure applied to the trigger point should not be hard enough to bruise, but should be strong enough to cause a sense of discomfort or tolerable pain. (This is sometimes described as a 'nice hurt'; that is, it is felt as a positive pain rather than a negative one).

Chilling and Stretching
This may be applied with either a piece of ice or a vapo-coolant spray.* Ideally the muscle in which the trigger (already identified and treated by pressure) lies should be placed in a position of stretch during the application of cold. Alternatively, the muscle

*Available at most chemist shops.

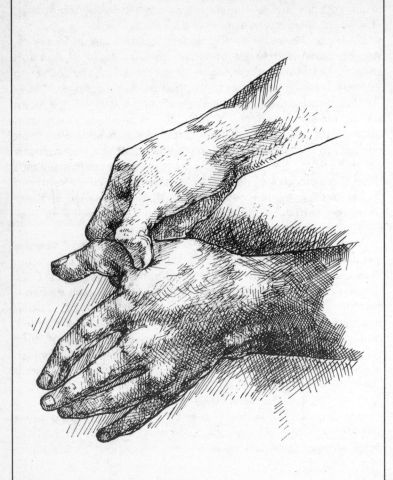

Thumb pressure technique applied to first interosseus muscle (see section 18).

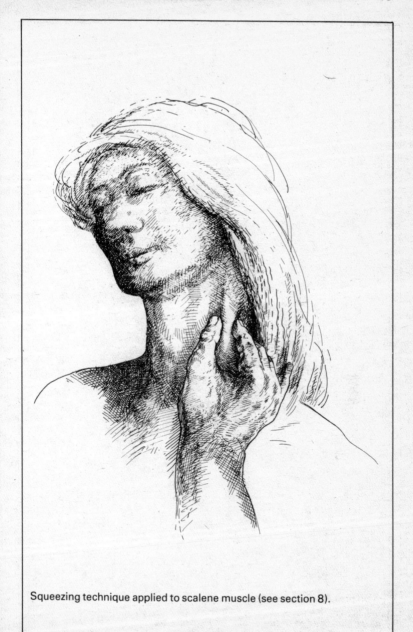

Squeezing technique applied to scalene muscle (see section 8).

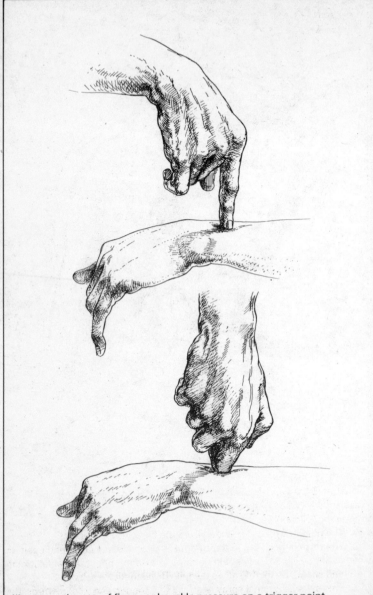

Illustrates the use of finger or knuckle pressure on a trigger point.

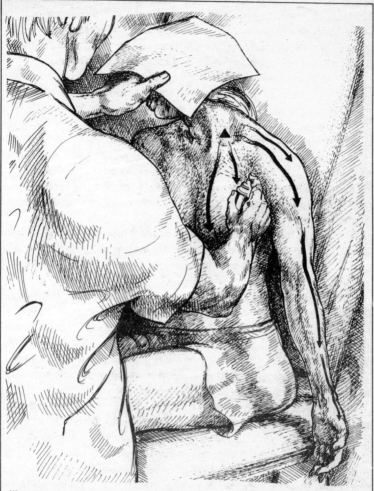

Illustrates the vapo-coolant (chilling) treatment of the trigger point in the scalenus muscles (see page 34).

Note the following points:

1. The patient's face is shielded from the spray.
2. The muscle involved in treatment is being held in a stretched position during chilling. This should be to the maximum of comfortable stretch and should be increased as the pain or restriction eases.
3. The sweeps of the spray start at the trigger and run towards the target (painful) areas. The sweeps are repeated several times.

should be stretched immediately after each chilling. If ice is used instead of the vapo-coolant spray, an edge of the ice should be employed and should trace the same pattern as followed by the spray (see illustration). Movement of the ice or the spray should be at a speed of between three and four inches per second.

If a spray is used it should be held eighteen to twenty-four inches from the point of application and the jet spray should be directed at the skin to meet it at an angle, not perpendicularly. The stream of vapo-coolant should start at the trigger point and the line of the sweep should be towards the target. Repeated sweeps should be made from the trigger to the target until the whole area (target as well as trigger) has been covered more than once. These sweeps of the spray (or glides of the ice) should be rhythmic – a few seconds on and a pause of a few seconds before beginning the next stroke.

Caution is required at this stage not to 'frost' the skin. If a deep aching or 'cold pain' results from the treatment, then a slightly longer gap is left between sweeps of the spray or application of the ice.

During the application of cold the muscle in which the trigger lies should be stretched. This should be gentle stretching and it should be maintained during each application. If there were restrictions in motion before treatment then periodically during the treatment the range of movement should be gently tested. This should always be within the limits of pain, as sudden over-stretching can cause more muscle spasm.

After several applications of cold, gentle pressure may be applied to the trigger to see if it still refers pain to the target area. If pain is no longer referred then cease treatment for that day. If pain is still referred then repeat the procedure once or twice. Altogether, ten minutes of intermittent spraying or icing and stretching may be needed. No more than this should be done on any one day, irrespective of continued pain. If pain is not substantially eased, then search for other triggers nearby as there can be several within a muscle, and the same techniques may be employed on these as well on a subsequent day.

If the use of pressure, chilling and stretching makes no marked difference to a particular pain then the causes probably lie elsewhere. Such causes might include joint or disc problems or systemic disease. Such causes, therefore, require appropriate advice from a qualified practitioner.

Diet

It is worth noting that a diet comprising at least fifty per cent raw food (salads, fruit etc.), and a minimum of refined carbohydrates and salt, and the avoiding of acid fruit and red meat, plus the addition of the following supplements will substantially reduce inflammatory muscular conditions and sensitivity to pain.

   Take Daily:
1 to 2g vitamin C.
100mg vitamin B_1 (thiamin).
1g daily calcium orotate (B_{13}-calcium)*
500mg daily magnesium orotate (B_{13}-magnesium).*
6 brewer's yeast tablets.

*United Kingdom source: Cantassium Company, 229 Putney Bridge Road, London SW 15.

INDEX OF SYMPTOMS

Note: The references given below are to Section numbers and not page numbers. For example: Abdomen, general relates to Section 23 on page 64.

1

STERNOMASTOID

The lower fibres originate from the upper end of the breast bone and insert into the mastoid bone, just behind the ear. Another branch originates from the inner third of the collar bone, inserting into the base of the skull.

Function

These muscles stabilize the neck and are the main muscles used to bend the neck forward. They also help to lift the collar bones and breast bone and are part of the breathing mechanism.

Trigger

A variety of trigger points can be found in these muscles after strain or injury. The main one is usually found in the belly of the muscle just below the level of the chin. This can best be found by gently squeezing the muscle between finger and thumb until the pain is caused in the target area.

Symptoms

Pain in the region of the ear, behind the ear, in the jaw, the throat and the frontal bones of the skull can all result from an active trigger in this muscle. Excessive or diminished skin function (such as dryness or oilyness or excessive sweating) on the face and head, sinus problems, allergies such as hay fever and difficulty in swallowing may all result from active triggers in this muscle.

Treatment

Pressure, applied by squeezing or pinching, followed by chilling and stretching of the muscle. Stretch by taking the head backwards and at the same time bending it and rotating it away from the treated side.

N.B. Shield eyes and ears from coolant spray.

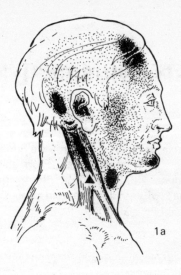

1a

Figures 1a) the sternomastoid trigger and target areas, 1b) treating the sternomastoid trigger, and 1c) the sternomastoid stretch.

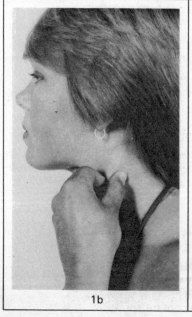

1b

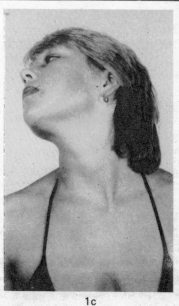

1c

2

SPLENIUS CAPITIS

The origins of this muscle are from the spines of the upper thoracic and lower cervical vertebrae. From there the fibres run upward and outward to insert, underneath the sternomastoid muscle (see page 20), into the mastoid process just behind the ear and at the base of the skull.

Function
This is another stabilizing muscle. When acting together with others, these two muscles (one either side) pull the head directly backwards. When acting alone they draw the head to one side and slightly rotate the face to the same side.

Trigger
This can be found just below the mastoid process by deep thumb or finger pressure. It is underneath the sternomastoid and requires penetrating pressure. The pain of pressing the trigger will give symptoms felt in the region on the top of the head directly above the ears.

Symptoms
The symptoms of an active trigger in this muscle will usually be pain and aching around the top of the head. Feelings of pressure or tingling or burning in this area are also common.

Treatment
Direct pressure onto the trigger and/or chilling, together with stretching, which is best achieved by taking the head as far forward as is possible and turning the face slightly away from the side being treated. This should be held for one to two minutes.

N.B. Shield eyes and ears from coolant spray.

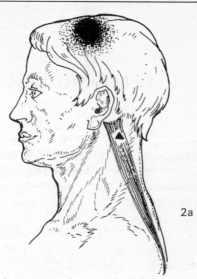

Figures 2a) the splenius capitis trigger and target areas, 2b) treating the splenius capitis trigger, and 2c) the splenius capitis stretch.

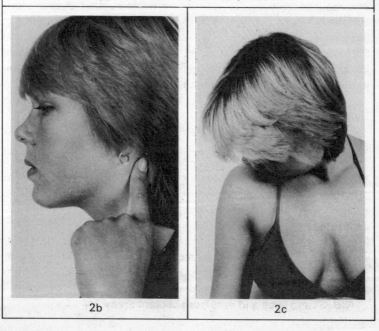

2b

2c

3

TEMPORALIS

This is a fan-shaped muscle situated at the side of the head. Its origins are on the temporal bone of the skull, its fibres converging to insert into the jaw.

Function
Its main function is to close the mouth. Its upper fibre can be felt above the temple when the teeth are being clenched, otherwise it is difficult to localize.

Trigger
A number of stresses can upset this muscle, such as uneven teeth, injuries to the face or jaw, distortion of the temporal bone through birth injury or dental problems (extractions etc.), tension induced by constant teeth clenching, as sometimes occurs in states of stress or anxiety etc. The trigger is found mid-way between the eye socket and the ear, above the cheek bone.

Symptoms
The main symptoms will be felt in the upper or lower jaw and teeth, above the eye and in the temporal area generally.

Treatment
Treatment is by direct pressure of a finger or thumb followed by chilling, from the trigger to the target, and stretching. The jaw should be held open as wide as possible and thrust slightly forward during the chilling. If necessary, a wedge of folded cardboard or some other material can be used to hold the mouth as widely open as possible during chilling and for a minute afterwards.

N.B. Shield eyes and ears from coolant spray.

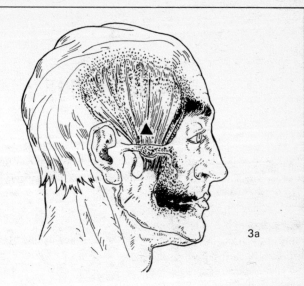

Figures 3a) the temporalis trigger and target areas, and 3b) treating the temporalis trigger.

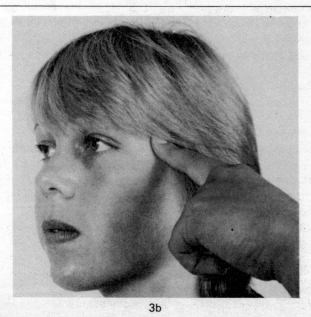

4

MASSETER

This is a square-shaped muscle consisting of three layers, one on the other. The fibres run from the cheek bone downward to the angle of the lower jaw.

Function
The main function is to raise the lower jaw. It can be easily felt in the cheek as the jaw is clenched.

Trigger
The main trigger will be found just above that part of the cheek bone that lies in front of the ear. The temple area is very sensitive at the best of times and probing with the thumb tip will locate the trigger which will refer pain anywhere on that side of the head or face, but primarily to the ear or teeth or gums, on the same side.

Symptoms
The pain can mimic toothache, ear-ache or generalized headache.

Treatment
Pressure applied to the trigger, followed by chilling of the trigger with sweeps towards the target area. Stretching can be applied during this treatment by propping the mouth comfortably open (to its maximum stretch), using a wedge of cardboard of some other material.

N.B. Shield eyes and ears from coolant spray and avoid inhaling fumes.

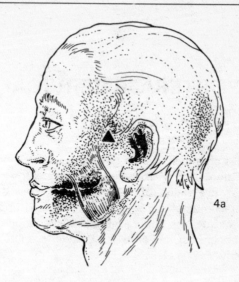

Figures 4a) the masseter trigger and target areas, and 4b) treating the masseter trigger.

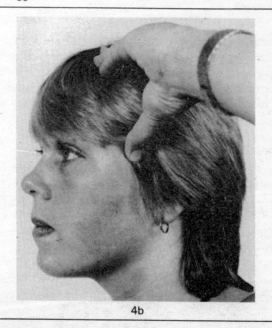

4b

5

POSTERIOR CERVICAL

These muscles are much like the guy ropes of a tent-pole, offering a degree of fine control to movement backwards of the head which may involve slight rotation and tilting. They arise from a variety of attachments in the lower cervical and upper thoracic region, such as the ribs and vertebral transverse processes, and insert in the upper neck and base of the skull.

Function
The main functions are to stabilize the head and to move it backwards or to rotate it backwards and to one side.

Trigger
These muscles tend to overlap each other. There are a number of areas where triggers may be found by deep palpation. The main trigger is just to the side of the spine, in the deep musculature of the neck, midway between the hair-line and the base of the neck, and will be found by deep pressure (thumb or finger) whilst the neck is in a resting position (either face down or seated).

Symptoms
Pain may be present at the base of the skull or on the inner aspect of the shoulder blade, or anywhere between these two areas. The muscles may be stiff and neck rotation restricted, together with difficulty in looking up and down.

Treatment
Pressure by thumb or finger followed by chilling treatment whilst the head is stretched forward (sitting with chin on chest, for example).

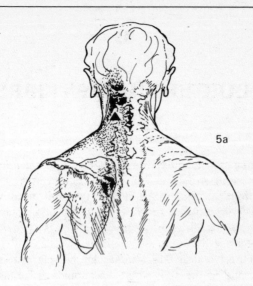

Figures 5a) the posterior cervical trigger and target areas, and 5b) treating the posterior cervical trigger.

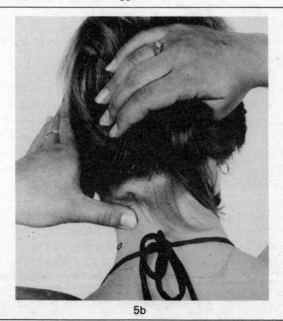

6

TRAPEZIUS (UPPER FIBRES)

The trapezius muscle is a flat triangular muscle, covering the back of the neck and shoulder. The upper fibres run downward and outwards from the base of the skull to the outer third of the collar bone.

Function
This upper part of the large, triangular muscle draws the head backwards and to the side when the shoulder is braced or fixed. Its other function is to stabilize or elevate the shoulder area during active use of the arm.

Trigger
This lies in the belly of the muscle, in the angle of the neck and shoulder. This can be found by pressure or squeezing.

Symptoms
Pain or numbness in the muscle itself, or at the angle of the jaw, the temporal area and the side of the head, may result from an active trigger in this muscle. This muscle is often sensitive with active triggers in conditions affecting the eyes and ears such as conjunctivitis, eye strain and defective hearing.

Treatment
By direct pressure or squeezing of the trigger between finger and thumb followed by chilling and stretching. Stretching is best achieved by tilting the head sideways away from the side of the trigger and pulling the shoulder, on that side, downwards.

N.B. Shield eyes and ears from coolant spray.

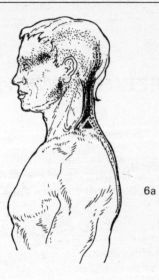

6a

Figures 6a) the upper trapezius trigger and target areas, 6b) treating the upper trapezius trigger, and 6c) the upper trapezius stretch.

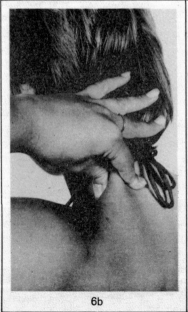

6b

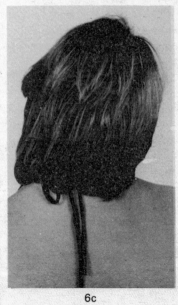

6c

7

TRAPEZIUS (LOWER FIBRES)

These fibres run upwards and outwards from the spinous processes of all the thoracic vertebrae to the inner end of the prominent ridge (spine) of the shoulder blade.

Function
This muscle stabilizes the shoulder blade and moves it to accommodate arm movement.

Trigger
There are often many sensitive points in this and the other muscles relating to the neck, some of which may refer pain to other areas. The main one in the lower trapezius lies between the spine and the lower edge of the shoulder blade (level of seventh or eighth thoracic vertebrae). It is found by simple pressure using finger or thumb.

Symptoms
Pain will be referred to the back of the neck, the upper shoulder and the back of the shoulder joint. There may be restrictions in shoulder and arm movement. These triggers are often active during colds and throat infections.

Treatment
Direct pressure followed by chilling and stretching. Stretch by raising the arm and stretching it upwards and away from the body whilst raising and carrying the shoulder blade outwards as far as possible.

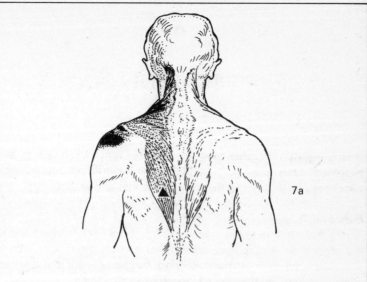

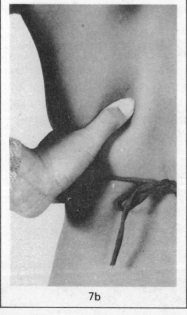
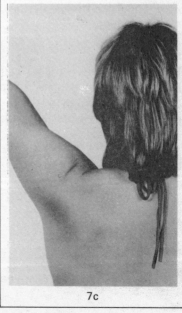

Figures 7a) the lower trapezius trigger and target areas, 7b) treating the lower trapezius trigger, and 7c) the lower trapezius stretch.

8

SCALENI

This is a group of three muscles, scalenus anterior, medium and posterior. They run from various attachments on the cervical vertebrae and insert into the front of the first and second ribs.

Function
Acting from below these muscles will pull the neck forward and to the same side. Acting from above, they elevate the first or second ribs. They are part of the stabilizing mechanism for the neck as well as having an effect on the breathing mechanism.

Trigger
At the angle of the neck above the collar bone almost directly in line with nipple.

Symptoms
Pain from an active trigger can be felt in the breast, upper arm, shoulder blade, shoulder, back of the upper arm, outer lower arm, or the back of the thumb, index finger and the half of the middle finger next to the index finger, all on the same side as the trigger.

Treatment
By direct pressure or squeezing (see drawing on page 13)—care should be taken in this region—followed by chilling and stretching. Stretch by rotating the head away from the active trigger and, at the same time, stretch the head backwards.

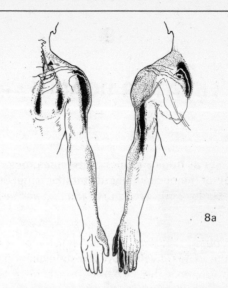

8a

Figures 8a) the scaleni trigger and target areas, and 8b) treating the scaleni trigger, and 8c) the scaleni stretch.

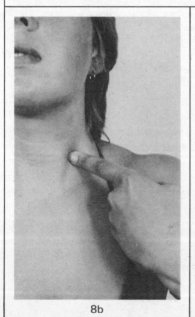

8b

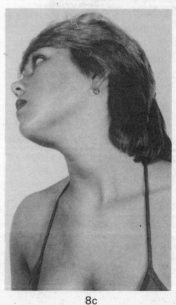

8c

9

LEVATOR SCAPULAE

This muscle has its origins on the transverse processes of the top four vertebrae of the neck. It inserts into the upper-inner border of the shoulder blade.

Function
Acting with other muscles, it steadies or moves the shoulder blade to accomodate movement of the shoulder and arm.

Trigger
Just above the inner-upper border of the shoulder blade.

Symptoms
Pain from this trigger may be felt on the side of the neck, the inner border of the shoulder blade and the back of the shoulder joint. There may also be a lop-sided carriage of the head if the muscle on one side is weaker, or tighter, than the other.

Treatment
Pressure, followed by chilling and stretching. Stretch by taking the head as far forward as possible whilst side bending and rotating it away from the side of the trigger.

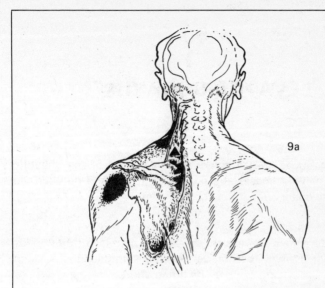

Figures 9a) the levator scapulae trigger and target areas, and 9b) treating the levator scapulae trigger.

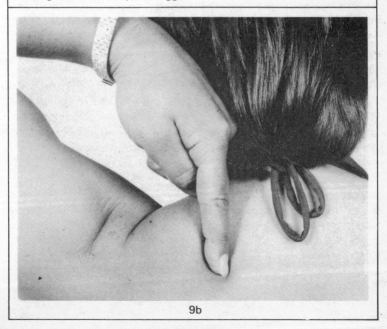

9b

10

SUPRASPINATUS

Originating above the prominent ridge (spine) of the shoulder blade in a hollow (fossa), the fibres run across and outwards to insert in the upper arm, at the shoulder joint.

Function
This muscle allows and assists the arm to be raised sideways by lifting out of the way the fibrous sac enclosing the shoulder joint and actually providing some of the lifting effort.

Trigger
This lies on the upper border of the shoulder blade about half way between the angle of the neck and the shoulder. It can be found by pressure.

Symptoms
An active trigger here will produce pain between the neck and shoulder and especially on the outer side of the shoulder joint itself running down the outer (thumb) side of the upper arm almost to the wrist. It can also produce difficulty in arm-raising. This area is often involved in so called 'frozen shoulder'.

Treatment
By pressure and chilling and stretching. Stretch by lifting the arm to its maximum, stretching it away from the body and gently rotating the upper arm externally (clockwise).

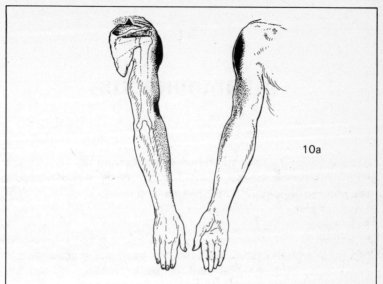

10a

Figures 10a) the supraspinatus trigger and target areas, and 10b) treating the supraspinatus trigger.

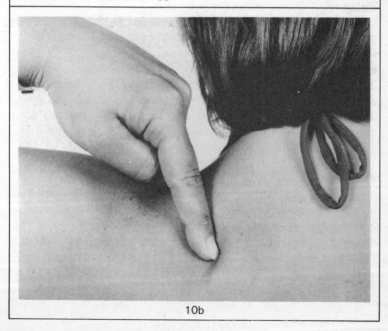

10b

11

INFRASPINATUS

This is a thick triangular muscle which arises from the inner border and the posterior surface of the shoulder blade, below its spine (the prominent ridge). It runs towards, and inserts into, the back of the upper arm.

Function
This muscle, with others, stabilizes the head of the upper arm in its position in the shoulder joint. It assists in lifting and rotating the arm outwards.

Trigger
Just below the spine of the shoulder blade (scapula) about one third of the distance from its inner border towards the shoulder.

Symptoms
Pain on the outer, upper arm and especially on the front of the shoulder joint running down the outer side and front of the arm to the hand. The two fingers adjacent to the thumb might be affected. This will often accompany difficulty in raising the arm and might be involved in a 'frozen shoulder' condition.

Treatment
By pressure and chilling and stretching. The arm should be raised and stretched away from the body whilst being internally rotated (anti-clockwise). If this is painful, it may be done by lying face downward on a bed with the arm hanging freely so that stretch is being applied and, at the same time, rotate the arm inwards.

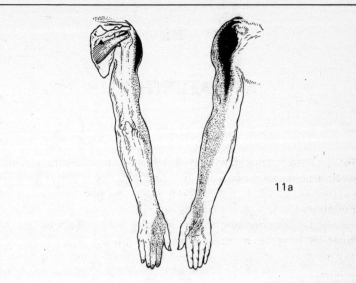

11a

Figures 11a) the infraspinatus trigger and target areas, 11b) treating the infraspinatus trigger, and 11c) the infraspinatus stretch.

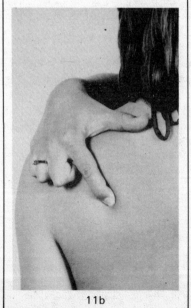

11b

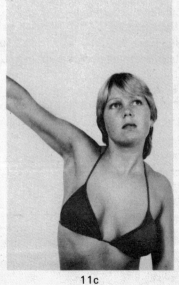

11c

12

DELTOID

This is a thick, triangular muscle which covers the shoulder joint. Its fibres are divided into anterior, posterior and middle fibres.

Function
Working independently, these different areas can raise the arm upwards, forwards or backwards, and rotate the arm.

Trigger
This lies in the front (anterior) fibres a little below the collar bone and one third the distance from the outer aspect. It is thus almost directly in line with the armpit. It is found by direct pressure.

Symptoms
Pain on the outer and front aspects of the shoulder joint and the upper arm often accompanied by difficulty in raising the arm.

Treatment
By pressure chilling and stretching. Stretch is achieved by taking the arm upwards and backwards as far as possible.

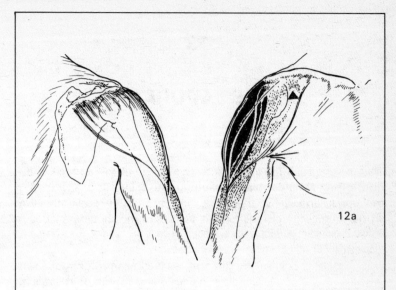

Figures 12a) the deltoid trigger and target areas, and 12b) treating the deltoid trigger.

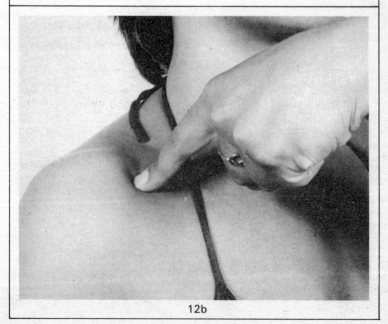

12b

13

SUBSCAPULARIS

This muscle runs from the outer two-thirds of the surface of the front of the shoulder blade, inserting into the front of the head of the upper arm. It is, therefore, only accessible under the arm where it crosses from the hidden aspects of the shoulder blade.

Function
This muscle aids in raising the arm as well as in rotating the arm inwards. It allows the shoulder blade to accommodate the raising of the arm above the head.

Trigger
In the armpit. It is found by pressing upwards and backwards and squeezing the area between the probing thumb and the index finger.

Symptoms
Pain under the arm, across the shoulder blade and especially at the back of the shoulder joint.

Treatment
By squeezing, chilling and stretching. Stretch by placing the hand behind the head and attempting to take the elbow as far forwards and upwards as possible.

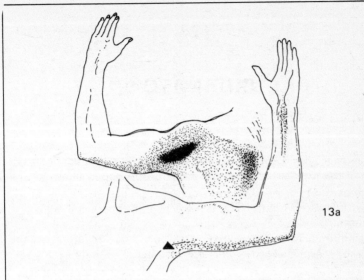

Figures 13a) the subscapularis trigger and target areas, and 13b) treating the subscapularis trigger.

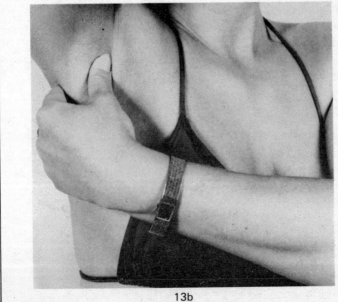

13b

14

SUPINATOR

This muscle runs from the lower, outer aspect of the upper arm to wind forwards to insert in the front of the upper aspect of the lower arm.

Function
This muscle rotates the lower arm outwards (to turn the palm upwards) especially when the arm is straight.

Trigger
This will be found near the outer aspect of the elbow crease by thumb or finger pressure. (This corresponds to the acupuncture point known as Colon 11).

Symptoms
Pain above the elbow and down the outer aspect of the forearm and especially on the back of the hand above the index finger.

Treatment
By pressure, chilling and stretching. Stretch is achieved by extending the arm and rotating the palm internally (anti-clockwise) as far as possible.

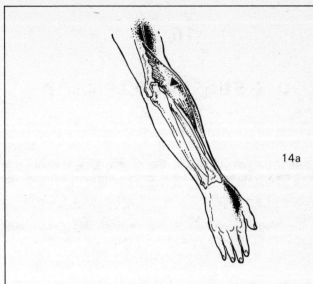

14a

Figures 14a) supinator trigger and target areas, and 14b) treating the supinator trigger.

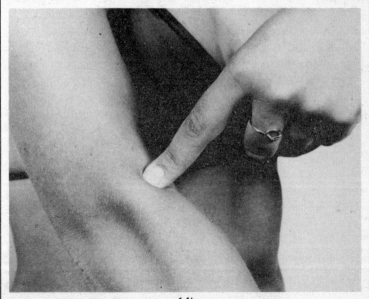

14b

15

MIDDLE FINGER EXTENSOR

Originating on the outer aspect of the elbow, this muscle runs downwards to insert, via four tendons, into the base of the fingers.

Function
To extend the fingers, especially the second and third, thus opening the hand.

Trigger
A little below the elbow joint, on the back of the arm, directly above the middle finger. Probing with the thumb will locate the trigger if it is active.

Symptoms
Pain on the back of the hand and down the arm. This can be of an aching nature and often accompanies difficulty in free wrist or hand movement.

Treatment
By pressure, chilling and stretching. Stretch is achieved by making a fist and flexing the wrist as far as possible.

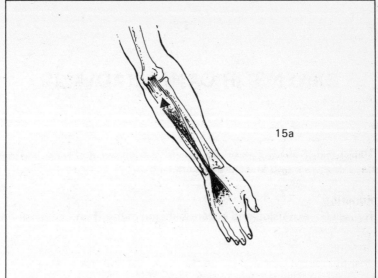

15a

Figures 15a) middle finger extensor trigger and target areas, and 15b) treating the middle finger extensor trigger.

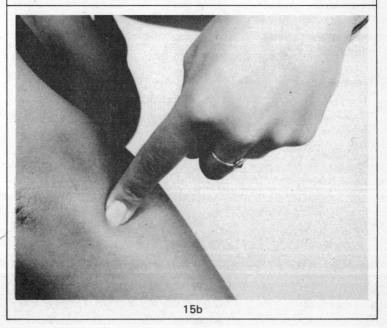

15b

16

EXTENSOR CARPI RADIALIS

This arises from the outer aspect of the elbow and runs to the base of the second and third fingers.

Function
To assist in extension and inward bending of the wrist.

Trigger
Just below the elbow joint on the outer aspect of arm above the index finger. This will be found by pressure.

Symptoms
Pain above the elbow joint and on the back of the hand. This often involves some difficulty in free use of the elbow and wrist and hand.

Treatment
Pressure, chilling and stretching. Stretch by straightening the arm, clenching the fist and bending the wrist outwards as far as possible.

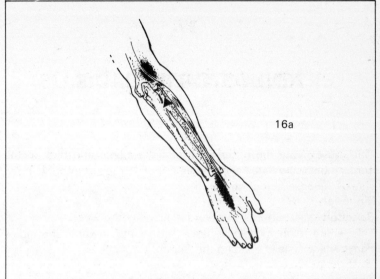

16a

Figures 16a) extensor carpi radialis trigger and target areas, and 16b) treating the extensor carpi radialis trigger.

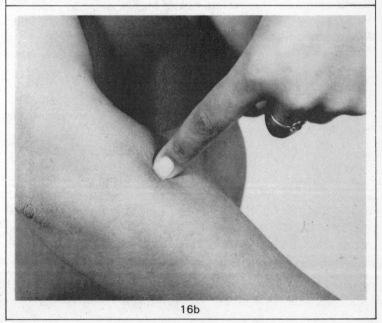

16b

17

ADDUCTOR POLLICIS

This muscle runs from the base of the second and third carpal bones (above the index and middle fingers) to insert into the inner side of the base of the thumb.

Function
This is the main muscle to draw the thumb towards the index finger and assists in bending the thumb.

Trigger
Between the thumb and index finger, slightly closer to the thumb than the trigger of the first interosseus muscle (see next page).

Symptoms
Pain and stiffness of the thumb – especially affecting the outer aspect of the base of the thumb.

Treatment
Pressure and chilling and stretching. Stretch by extending the thumb (hitch-hiking position) to its maximum.

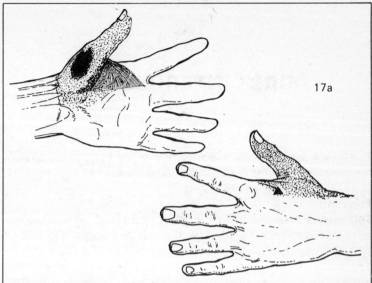

Figures 17a) adductor pollicis trigger and target areas, and 17b) treating the adductor pollicis trigger.

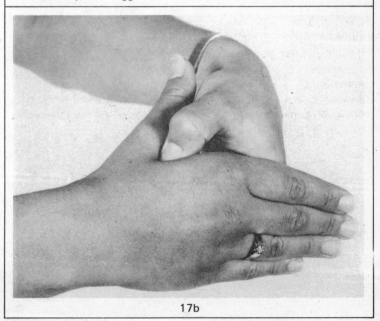

17b

18

FIRST INTEROSSEUS

This runs from the inner, upper surface of the bone at the base of the thumb to the thumb side of the index finger.

Function
This muscle helps to bend the index finger and takes it across, towards the thumb when the hand is stretched open.

Trigger
In the muscle between the thumb and index finger. (This corresponds to the acupuncture point known as Hoku or Colon 4).

Symptoms
Pain and stiffness affecting the palm and back of the hand especially on the thumb side of the index finger.

Treatment
Pressure, chilling and stretching. Stretch is achieved by pointing the index finger whilst the thumb is taken as far outward as comfortably possible.

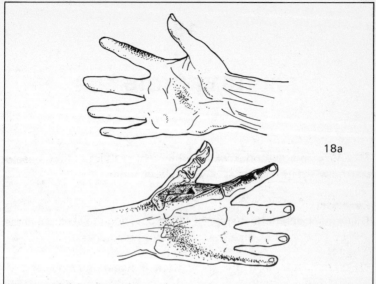

Figures 18a) first interosseus trigger and target areas, and 18b) treating the interosseus trigger.

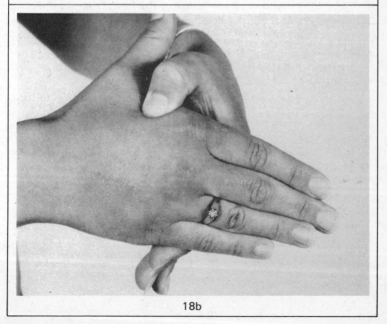

18b

19

STERNALIS

This is a rudimentary muscle which is in effect a thin layer of muscular tissue covering the breast bone (sternum).

Function
It has no apparent function other than covering the sternum.

Trigger
On the breast bone, a little above a line between the nipples.

Symptoms
Pain on the breast bone, at the base of the throat, across the collar bones and down the inner sides of the upper arms.

Treatment
By pressure and chilling.

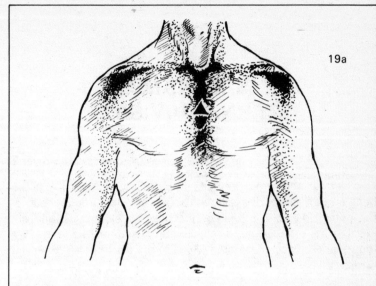

Figures 19a) sternalis trigger and target areas, and 19b) treating the sternalis trigger.

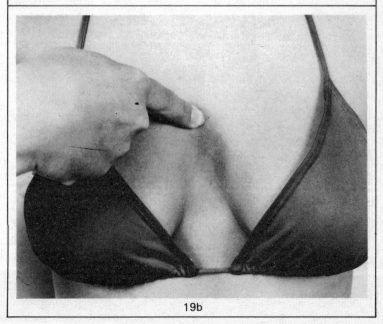

19b

20

PECTORALIS MAJOR (STERNAL DIVISION)

This part of the large triangular muscle arises from the breast bone and the upper ribs and runs across and upwards to insert on the outer side of the upper arm. These fibres curve round and envelop the other pectoral muscle fibres (see next page) to form the rounded muscular bundle which forms the front of the armpit (axilla).

Function
This part of the muscle pulls the arm towards and across the vertical mid-line of the body, as well as helping to lift and rotate it inwards.

Trigger
This can be found in the fold of muscle in front of the armpit by squeezing or pressure.

Symptoms
Pain in the upper chest muscles, especially just to the side of the nipple, running towards the armpit. This muscle is often tense and painful in stress conditions.

Treatment
Pressure via squeezing, chilling and stretching. Stretch by taking the arm up, back and rotating it outwards as far as possible.

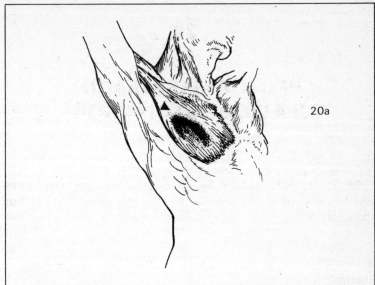

20a

Figures 20a) pectoralis major (sternal division) trigger and target areas, and 20b) treating the pectoralis major (sternal) trigger.

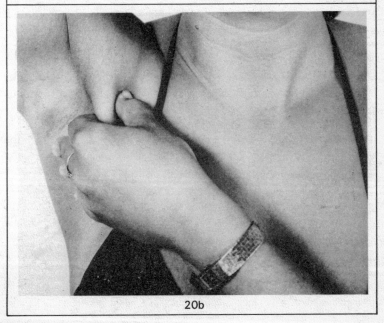

20b

21

PECTORALIS MAJOR (CLAVICULAR DIVISION)

This part of this fan-shaped muscle extends from the inner half of the collar bone, across and slightly downwards and inserts into the upper arm.

Function
These fibres aid in bending and raising the upper arm at the shoulder.

Trigger
Between the collar bone and the nipple – this can be located by pressure.

Symptoms
Pain in the breast area radiating towards the arm and down the inner side of the arm. This area is often involved in stress and emotional conditions.

Treatment
By pressure, chilling and stretching. Stretch by turning and stretching the arm outwards and away from the body.

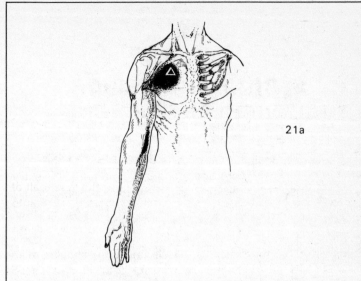

21a

Figures 21a) pectoralis major (clavicular division) trigger and target areas, and 21b) treating the pectoralis major (clavicular) trigger.

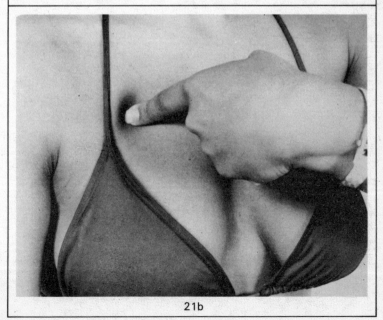

21b

22

SERRATUS ANTERIOR

These muscles originate from the outer surface of the upper border of the ribs. The fibres intermingle and run round the side of the body to insert onto the surface of the shoulder blade closest to the spine.

Function
Acting with other muscles, this muscle draws the shoulder blade forwards. It is the main muscle concerned in all pushing and punching movements, and with the movement of the shoulder blade when the arm is raised above the head.

Trigger
Just below and slightly posterior to the front of the armpit.

Symptoms
Pain in the upper, outer aspect of the chest, under the arm and on the lower, inner aspect of the shoulder blade. Some discomfort may radiate down the inner arm to the palm of the hand.

Treatment
Pressure, chilling and stretching. Stretch by pulling the shoulder blade as close to the spine as possible whilst the arm is twisted behind the back so that the hand is reaching for the opposite shoulder blade.

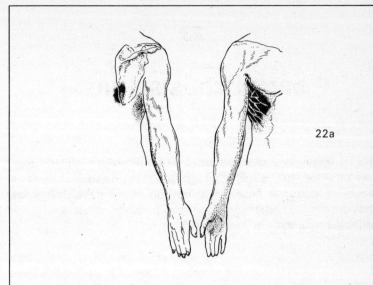

Figures 22a) serratus anterior trigger and target areas, and 22b) treating the serratus anterior trigger.

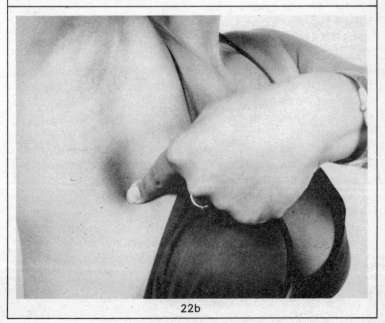

22b

23

MULTIFIDUS SPINAE

This muscle is in reality a series of muscular strips which lie deep in the muscles of the back and which fill the groove at the side of the spine from the base up to the top of the neck. The strips (fasciculi) vary in length and connect the point of origin with the vertebrae two, three or even four above it.

Function
These are mainly postural muscles. They control stability and movement of the spinal joints thus aiding the action of the larger back muscles. Depending upon which combination of these are involved, they can produce some back-bending, side-bending and rotatory movements.

Trigger
There are many myofascial triggers in these muscles, but the main ones are (1) just above the waist close to the spine and (2) near to the base of the spine.

Symptoms
Pain local to the trigger as well as some pain referred to the abdomen on the same side and at the same level. Such triggers are often associated with stiffness and spasm of the back.

Treatment
Pressure, chilling and stretching. Stretch by carefully bending forward, side-bending and rotating away from the side of pain.

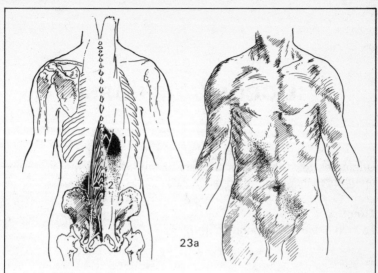

Figures 23a) multifidus spinae trigger and target areas, 23b) treating the upper multifidus spinae trigger, and 23c) treating the lower multifidus spinae trigger.

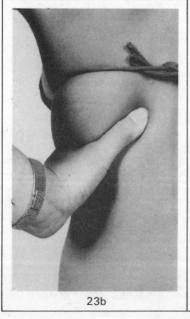

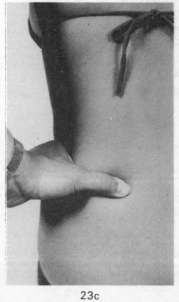

24

ILIOCOSTALIS DORSI

Originates from the upper borders of the lower six ribs and runs upwards to insert in the upper six ribs.

Function
To help in backward bending of the spine.

Trigger
In line with the inner border of the shoulder blade at the level of the eighth or ninth rib.

Symptoms
Pain in the region of the trigger radiating round to the side, as well as pain in the lower abdomen on the same side.

Treatment
Pressure, chilling and stretching. Stretch by carefully bending forwards and to the side opposite the pain.

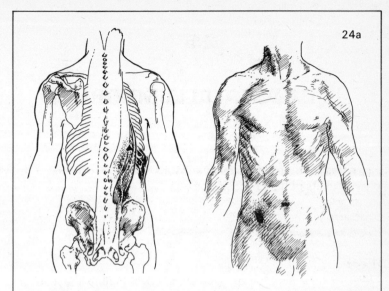

Figures 24a) iliocostalis dorsi trigger and target areas, and 24b) treating the iliocostalis dorsi trigger.

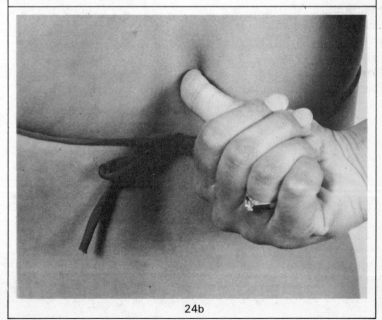

24b

25

ILIOCOSTALIS LUMBORUM

Originates from the pelvic crest and runs upwards to insert on the lower aspects of the lower six ribs.

Function
To aid in backward bending of the spine.

Trigger
A little to the side of the spine below the twelfth rib.

Symptom
Pain locally and below the trigger running down to the base of the spine and the buttock.

Treatment
Deep pressure, chilling and stretching. Stretch by carefully bending forward and to the opposite side of the pain.

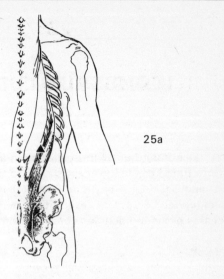

25a

Figures 25a) iliocostalis lumborum trigger and target areas, and 25b) treating the iliocostalis lumborum trigger.

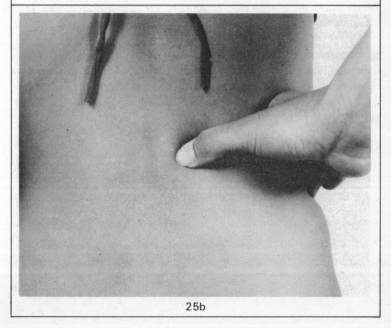

25b

26

LONGISSIMUS DORSI

This is part of a group of muscles known as the erector spinae. It arises from the crest of the pelvis and sacrum and the lower spinal joints and as it runs upwards some of its fibres attach to the lumbar vertebrae, others insert into the tips of the transverse processes of the thoracic vertebrae and into the lower ten ribs.

Function
The action is to bend the spine backwards and to the side.

Trigger
There are many myofascial triggers in these spinal muscles. Two major ones are at the level of the eighth and ninth ribs.

Symptoms
If at the level of the eighth rib, pain will extend downwards to the lumbar area, the base of the spine and the buttock. If at the level of the ninth rib, pain will extend downwards to the crest of the pelvis.

Treatment
Deep pressure, chilling and stretching. Stretch by carefully bending forward and to the side opposite the pain.

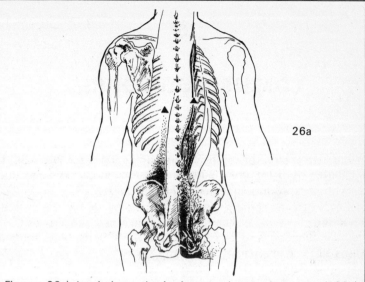

26a

Figures 26a) longissimus dorsi trigger and target areas, and 26b) treating the longissimus dorsi trigger.

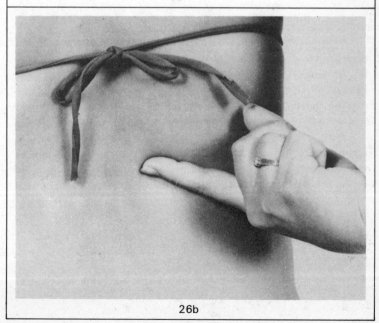

26b

27

GLUTEUS MEDIUS

A broad muscle which lies on the outer side of the pelvis. It originates from the outer surface of the crest of the pelvis and runs down to insert into the side of the upper leg.

Function
Its main function is to raise the leg sideways. Some of its anterior fibres assist in internal rotation of the leg.

Trigger
Just below the highest point of the crest of the pelvis.

Symptoms
Pain running from just to the side of the spine, along the crest of the pelvis and over the hip joint, as well as in the buttock.

Treatment
Pressure, chilling and stretching. Stretch by carrying the leg across the vertical mid-line of the body whilst rotating it outwards.

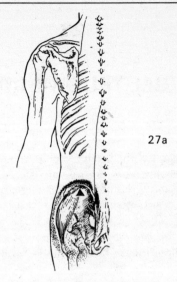

27a

Figures 27a) gluteus medius trigger and target areas, and 27b) treating the gluteus medius trigger.

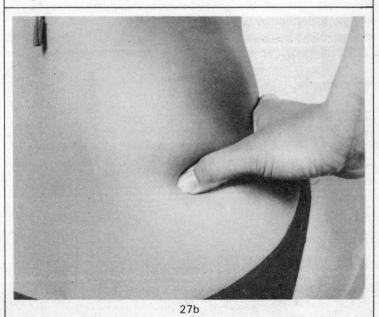

27b

28

GLUTEUS MINIMUS

This is the smallest of the three glutei muscles. It lies at the side of the pelvis (under the gluteus medius — see page 72). It originates from the upper, outer rim of the pelvis (crest of the ilium) and runs downwards to insert into the front, outer surface of the upper leg.

Function
The action of this muscle is to assist in raising the leg sideways and in its internal rotation.

Triggers
This is an extremely sensitive area and a number of myofascial triggers may be found there. The two main ones are (1) posterior gluteus minimus trigger, which lies at the back of the muscle, and (2) lateral gluteus minimus trigger, which lies between the outer rim of the pelvic bone and the hip joint (two-thirds of the way upwards).

Symptoms
Trigger (1) will produce pain locally, over the muscle, in the buttock, down the back of the thigh and into the calf. Trigger (2) will produce pain in the buttock, down the side of the thigh and outer aspect of the lower leg.

These pains can be mistaken for sciatic pain or hip joint disease.

Treatment
Pressure (to the level of pain tolerance), chilling and stretching. Stretch by rotating the leg outwards and carrying it across the other leg, whilst lying face upwards.

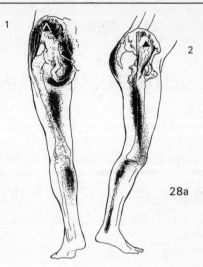

Figures 28a) gluteus minimus trigger and target areas, 28b) treating the gluteus minimus trigger 1, and 28c) treating the gluteus minimus trigger 2.

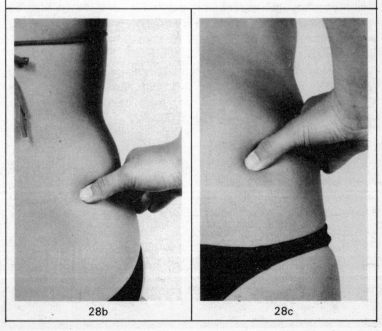

29

ADDUCTOR LONGUS

This triangular muscle extends from the front of the pubic bone (symphysis pubis), running downwards and outwards to insert into the middle third of the inner side of the thigh bone.

Function
This muscle aids in lifting the upper leg and is largely responsible for adduction (that is, it brings the leg inwards and across the vertical mid-line of the body).

Triggers
One trigger lies about one third of the way down, in the belly of the muscle. The other lies half-way down on its upper surface.

Symptoms
The first trigger produces pain in the muscle itself and the second produces pain in the front of the hip joint, down the inside of the thigh and above the inside of the knee extending to the upper inner calf. This can mimic hip joint pain.

Treatment
Pressure, chilling and stretching. Stretch by taking the leg sideways as far as possible and stretching it backwards, or by sitting with the heel of the affected leg resting on the opposite knee whilst the affected knee is allowed to stretch outwards.

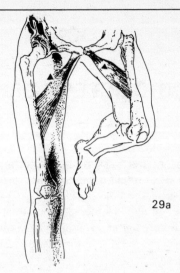

29a

Figures 29a) adductor longus trigger and target areas, 29b) treating the adductor longus (upper) trigger, and 29c) treating the adductor longus (lower) trigger.

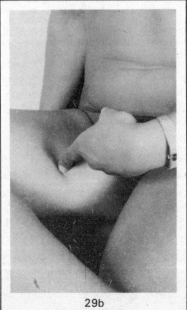

29b

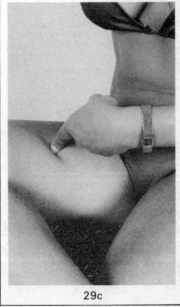

29c

30

BICEPS FEMORIS

This muscle lies at the back of the thigh and arises from two heads. The long head runs from the lower margin of the pelvis and the short head from the upper thigh bone. They run downwards, forming what is known as the lateral hamstring, to eventually insert into the outer, upper aspects of the tibia and fibula (shin bones).

Function
The muscle extends the upper leg, i.e. it helps to take it backwards. It is mainly effective in this respect when the knee is straight. The long head runs across the sciatic nerve and can impinge upon it.

Trigger
On the inner aspect of the belly of the long head, where it joins with another of the muscles of the back of the leg. The trigger is almost central, in that it lies half-way between the knee crease and the buttock crease. It corresponds to Bladder Point 51 in acupuncture.

Symptoms
Pain in the lower thigh, behind the knee joint and in the upper calf.

Treatment
Pressure and chilling and stretching. Stretch by keeping the knee straight and raising the leg forwards and upwards to its tolerable limit.

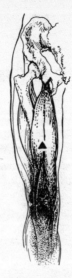

30a

Figures 30a) biceps femoris trigger and target areas, and 30b) treating the biceps femoris trigger.

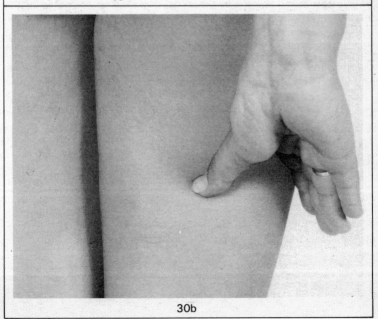

30b

31

VASTUS MEDIALIS

This muscle lies on the inner aspect of the thigh. It arises from the inner upper thigh bone and runs downwards and forwards to insert into the inner side of the knee cap (patella), and by ligament to the tibia.

Function
This aids in straightening of the knee joint and helps to stabilize the joint.

Trigger
Above the inner margin of the knee cap on the inner side of the thigh.

Symptoms
Pain on the knee cap and around the front of the joint, especially above it. This can seem like a pain in the knee joint.

Treatment
Pressure and chilling and stretching. Stretch by bending the knee to its fullest.

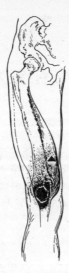

31a

Figures 31a) vastus medialis trigger and target areas, and 31b) treating the vastus medialis trigger.

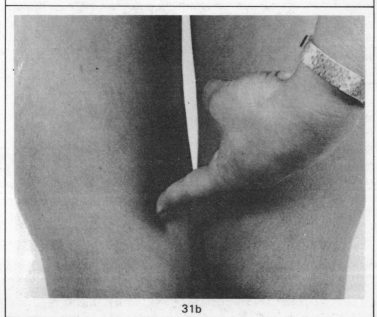

31b

32

GASTROCNEMIUS

This muscle forms the greater part of the calf. It rises by two heads from the lower aspect of the upper bone of the leg, the femur. These run down the back of the calf where they join a strong tendon which inserts into the back of the heel. (This is the Achilles tendon).

Function
With other muscles it flexes the foot and bends the knee. It provides a major part of the motive force in walking, running and jumping.

Trigger
This is found just above the belly of the muscle, slightly towards the inner aspect.

Symptoms
Pain on the inner side of the calf running downward to the heel. Also pain under the heel and instep.

Treatment
Pressure, chilling and stretching. Stretch by straightening the leg and drawing the top of the foot towards the knee.

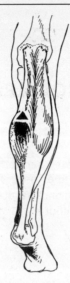

32a

Figures 32a) gastrocnemius trigger and target areas, and 32b) treating the gastrocnemius trigger.

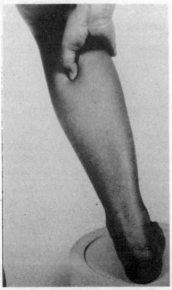

32b

33

SOLEUS

This is a broad, flat muscle lying in front of gastrocnemius. It arises from the back and outer aspect of the upper part of the lower leg, just below the knee. Insertion is into the heel bone by attachment to the Achilles tendon.

Function
Flexion of the foot, i.e. pointing the toes. (This is known as plantar-flexion.)

Trigger
Just above Achilles tendon where the belly of the muscle begins.

Symptoms
Pain in the heel and in the tendon running down to it.

Treatment
By pressure, chilling and stretching. Straightening the leg and drawing the top of the foot towards the knee.

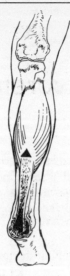

33a

Figures 33a) soleus trigger and target areas, and 33b) treating the soleus trigger.

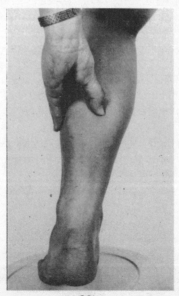

33b

34

EXTENSOR DIGITORUM LONGUS

This lies on the outer side of the front of the lower leg. It arises from the outer, upper aspect of the front shin bone (tibia) and from the front of the upper three-quarters of the posterior shin bone (fibula). It runs down to insert on the top of the outer four toes.

Function
This muscle has specific action on the toes, straightening them; of the ankle, flexing it; and on the foot, drawing to the top of the foot towards the knee and carrying it outwards.

Trigger
A quarter of the way down the outer side of the front of the lower leg.

Symptoms
Pain on the top of the foot and running down the outer side of the lower leg.

Treatment
Pressure, chilling and stretching. Stretch by plantar-flexion i.e. point the foot and bend the toes.

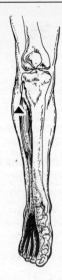

34a

Figures 34a) extensor digitorum longus trigger and target areas, and 34b) treating the extensor digitorum longus trigger.

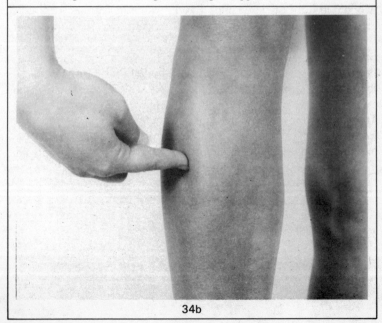

34b

35

TIBIALIS ANTICUS

This muscle runs down the front of the outer side of the lower leg and crosses to run towards the inner side of the foot, where it inserts under the foot at the head of the big toe.

Function
This muscle pulls the top of the foot up towards the knee and also inverts it. It also lifts and rotates the big toe.

Trigger
This lies just to the outer side of the shin bone a quarter of the way down from the knee joint. (It approximates Stomach Point 36 in acupuncture).

Symptoms
Pain down the front of the shin and the inner and front aspect of the foot and especially the big toe.

Treatment
Pressure, chilling and stretching. Stretch by pointing the toes and curling them under.

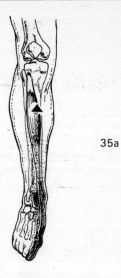

35a

Figures 35a) tibialis anticus trigger and target areas, and 35b) treating the tibialis anticus trigger.

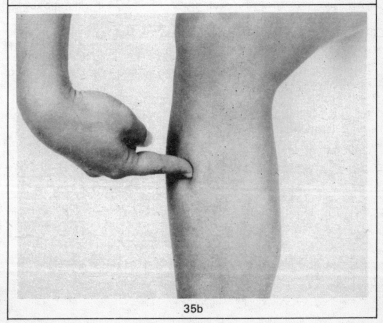

35b

36

PERONEUS LONGUS

This muscle runs down the side of the lower leg from origins below the knee on the shin bones (tibia and the fibula). It runs under the instep and across to insert at the head of the big toe.

Function
This muscle flexes the foot at the ankle and turns the foot outwards and bends it forwards.

Trigger
Just in front of and below the head of the fibula, the posterior shin bone. (This corresponds to Gall Bladder Point 34 in acupuncture).

Symptoms
Pain on the outer side of the back of the lower leg, running around the outside of the ankle.

Treatment
Pressure, chilling and stretching. Stretch by pointing the foot and turning it inwards.

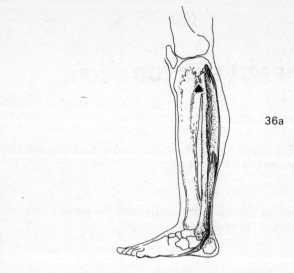

36a

Figures 36a) peroneus longus trigger and target areas, and 36b) treating the peroneus longus trigger.

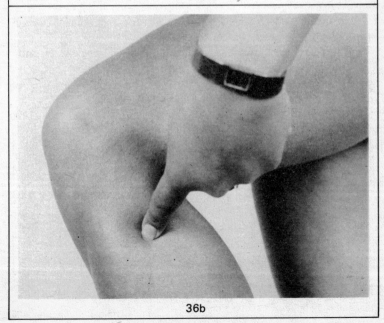

36b

ABDUCTOR HALLUCIS

This muscle lies along the inner border of the foot. It originates mainly from the base of the heel and inserts into the big toe.

Function
To assist in the weight-bearing activities and contributes towards the maintenance of the feet arches.

Trigger
On the inside of the foot, below and in front of the ankle.

Symptom
Pain is under and to the side of the big toe (especially 'bunion' type of pain).

Treatment
Pressure, chilling and stretching. Stretch by bringing the big toe up and towards the vertical mid-line of the body.

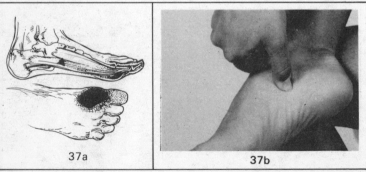

37a

37b

Figures 37a) abductor hallucis trigger and target areas, and 37b) treating the abductor hallucis trigger.

SHORT EXTENSORS

This thin muscle originates on the upper, outer surface of the ankle and runs over the top of the foot to insert via four tendons into the top of the big toe and the next three toes.

Function
To extend the toes in which it inserts.

Trigger
On the top of the foot just below the ankle to the outer side.

Symptoms
Locally to the trigger and over to top outer side of the foot.

Treatment
Pressure, chilling and stretching. Stretch by curling the toes.

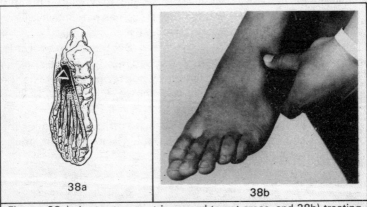

38a

38b

Figures 38a) short extensors trigger and target areas, and 38b) treating the short extensors trigger.

39

ABDOMINAL TRIGGER POINTS

A number of researchers have noted the existence of trigger points in the abdominal region. Dr R. Gutstein described triggers (see Figure 39) which, when treated successfully, removed a host of symptoms ranging from excessive or poor appetite to nervous vomiting, flatulence and loose bowels. Dr Janet Travel (once President Kennedy's personal physician) has described similar points which were related to pain, as well as nervous conditions such as hysteria. Trigger points are found in any of the abdominal muscles and the illustration only gives examples of commonly found points. When treated by pressure and chilling and stretching, these and other symptoms may be considerably improved. Of course there may be other factors such as dietary errors and emotional problems involved in these conditions, and these should also be dealt with if long-term improvements are to be gained. However, the removal of these triggers can be a marvellous first aid measure and can start the process of recovery, for if left untreated these triggers can maintain a condition such as nervous vomiting, even when dietary considerations have been dealt with.

In order to localize these points the patient lies face upwards, knees bent. The muscles are probed for sensitive points. Treatment is by pressure, delivered by squeezing or pressing the point, fairly strongly, for up to two minutes, followed by chilling and stretching.

Stretch by lying face upwards with a soft cushion under the low back. Rest in this position whilst doing slow, deep breathing for some minutes after chilling.

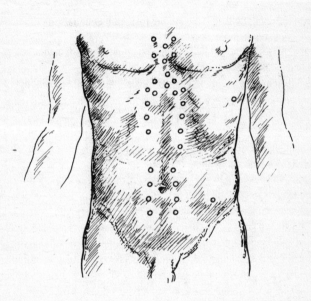

Figure 39. Gutstein's myodysneuric points.

INDEX OF MUSCLES